The ~~Official~~ V.I.P.

VERY IMPORTANT PATIENT

Handbook

V.I.P. Hospital Productions

ISBN: 978-1-63110-136-6
LCCN: 2015934987

A Product of V.I.P. Hospital Productions
www.viphospitalproductions.org

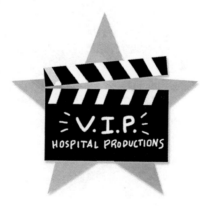

Find us on Facebook and follow us on
Twitter @viphospitalprod

Being a V.I.P.* means spending time at the Hotel Hospitalle.

It may not have a red carpet, but those who stay here often wear gowns.

People may be obsessed with taking your picture.

Or hoping your heart beats for them.

But it's a place where your entourage sees to your every need.

And your fans cheer you on!

GET WELL SOON

*VERY IMPORTANT PATIENT

HOW TO USE THE ~~OFFICIAL~~
V.I.P. HANDBOOK

Write, DRAW, Create, and use this
handbook as needed for:

- Communicating
- Venting
- Laughing
- Sharing
- Philosophizing
- Day Dreaming
- Hoping
- Pondering
- Interacting
- Playing
- Exploring
- Imagining
- Healing
- Bonding
- Expressing
- Empowering
- Time-passing
- Fun and gaming

NO RESTRICTIONS

MEMBERS OF MY FAN CLUB ARE: (friends, family, visitors)

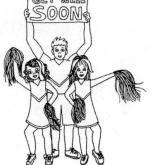

MEMBERS OF MY ENTOURAGE ARE: (doctors, nurses, other people at the hospital)

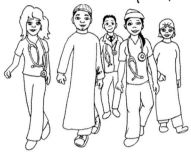

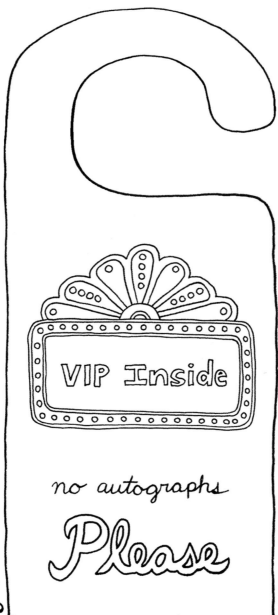

Hang me on your door
Make your own
Door Sign:

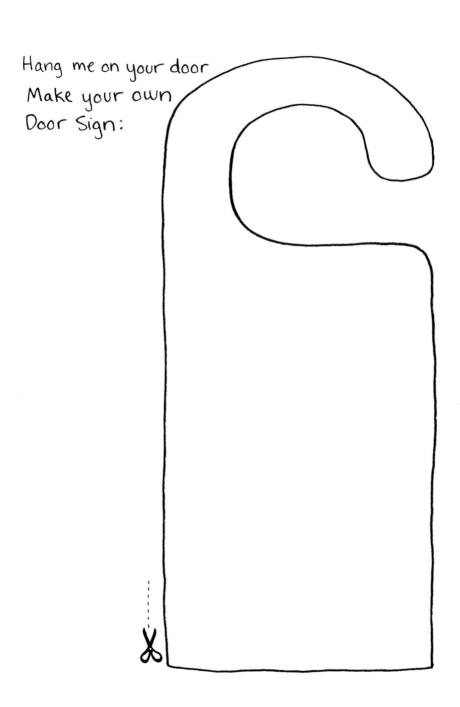

"THE INSIDE STORY ON MY V.I.P. LIFE":

My favorite TV shows are:

Favorite movies:

Favorite bands/musicians:

Favorite books/things to read:

Favorite clothing/brands:

Favorite places to hang out:

Favorite foods:

Favorite sports teams:

Favorite subject in school:

YOUR V.I.P. SUITE

DRAW A FLOOR PLAN OF YOUR ROOM OR MAYBE EVEN THE WHOLE HOSPITAL (THE REAL OR YOUR OWN IMPROVED VERSION)

SCAVENGER HUNT #1
Getting to know the Hotel Hospitalle:

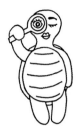

- Number of rooms on your floor:

- Approximate size of your room in square feet:

- Number of blue items in your bathroom:
    - List them:

- Five different types of doctors who work at your hospital:

- Find things in your room that begin with the letter "S":

- The name of the head nurse on your floor:

- The name of a doctor who visits your room today:

- The name of a Child Life worker or volunteer:

- Someone who worked here for 20+ years:

3 other people you encounter today at the hospital

1. What is their job title?
    What does it really mean?

2. What is their job title?
    What does it really mean?

3. What is their job title?
    What does it really mean?

WHAT'S UP DOC?

(Tear out as needed and find more memos in the back of the book).

- -

MEMOS FOR MY ENTOURAGE

For my:
- ☐ Doctor
- ☐ Nurse
- ☐ Other; _____
- _____

Concerning:
- ☐ Questions I have
- ☐ Comments
- ☐ Ideas
- ☐ Problems
- ☐ Something else

- -

MEMOS FOR MY ENTOURAGE

For my:
- ☐ Doctor
- ☐ Nurse
- ☐ Other; _____
- _____

Concerning:
- ☐ Questions I have
- ☐ Comments
- ☐ Ideas
- ☐ Problems
- ☐ Something else

PAGE OF GOOD THOUGHTS

WORDS TO IMPRESS #1:

"This new soap is making my epidermis very soft!"

Rhinorrea: (rhy nor **ree** ah) a runny nose.

Patella: (puh **tell** ah) knee cap.

Axilla: (ag **zil** ah) armpit.

Epidermis: (ep i **dur** mis) skin.

Pyrexia: (pie **wrek** see ah) fever.

Syncope: (sing kuh pee) faint.

Borborygmi: (bor buh **rig** my) the rumbling sounds in your tummy!

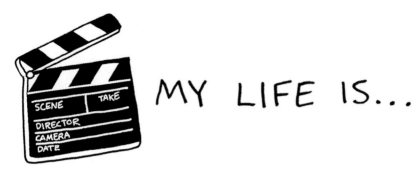 MY LIFE IS...

A sitcom because:

A drama because:

Make your own Comic:

TRUTH...

2 TRUTHS AND A LIE COMPETITION: YOU vs. Your ENTOURAGE

THE RULES: MAKE 3 STATEMENTS ABOUT YOURSELF—2 ARE TRUE AND ONE WILL BE A LIE. SEE IF A MEMBER FROM YOUR ENTOURAGE CAN GUESS THE LIE. THEN SWITCH ROLES AND IT'S YOUR TURN TO GUESS!

Scoreboard:

	Round #1 (They guess)	Round #2 (I guess)
Me vs. _____ :		
Me vs. _____ :		
Me vs. _____ :		

√ = Got it right!

X = Got it wrong

OR DARE!

- [ ] Ask a member of your entourage: "Do you have holes in your underwear?" When they tell you, "No, of course not!" say, "That's incredible! How do you get your legs in them?"

Convince a member of your entourage that...

- [ ] You are related to a celebrity.

- [ ] Your first name is really something else.

- [ ] It's a different day of the week.

- [ ] There's a weird purple spot on your wall.

DESTROY

this page when you're

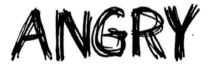

Practice your *Autograph*:

Write your name BIG:

Write your name little:

Write your name backwards:

Write your name in a circle:

Write your name with your eyes closed:

Write your name using your favorite color:

Write your fancy signature:

V. I. P. VICTORIES
I am proud of...

PAGE OF DOODLES

READ SOMEONE'S MIND

Ask someone to think of
a number between 1 and 10.

Tell them to multiply their
number by 2...

Then add 10...

Then divide by 2...

Finally, tell them to subtract
their ORIGINAL NUMBER...

Now you can amaze them!
Tell them the number they
are left with is 5!
(It will always be 5).

THINGS I WISH MY FRIENDS KNEW ABOUT MY V.I.P. LIFE:

SCAVENGER HUNT #2

Complete by yourself or tear in half
and complete with a friend!

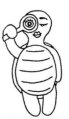

- -

Collect autographs from a member OF YOUR
ENTOURAGE WHO...

Has been to the statue of liberty _____
Plays video games _____
Speaks more than one language _____
Likes the same sports team as you _____
Has read all the Hunger Games books _____
Has gone sky-diving _____
Has been to a rock concert _____
Has met a celebrity _____
Has a cat _____
Has over 500 Facebook friends _____

- -

Collect autographs from a member OF YOUR
ENTOURAGE WHO...

Has been to the Eiffel Tower _____
Was born in another country _____
Likes rollercoasters _____
Has been in a school play _____
Knows how to surf _____
Has an iPhone _____
Can juggle _____
Can do an impression of a celebrity _____
Has a dog _____
Plays the guitar _____

Map out the things that take up space in your brain:

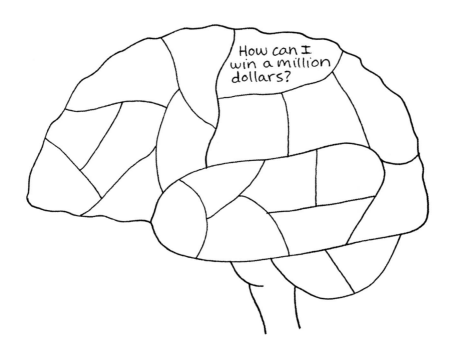

TEST YOUR ENTOURAGE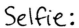

See if your entourage
can define the
following words and phrases.

Selfie:
ROTFL:
Photobomb:
Meme:
Hashtag:
Bae:
Biffle:
SMH:
#MCM:
#TBT:
YOLO:
LOL:
BRB:
TTYL:
GIF:
Emoji:

Hospital Hollywood

Make medical versions of movie titles!
Example: Harry Potter and the Half-Blood
pressure prince

Collect ideas from your entourage and fan club!

Draw the movie poster for one of these new films:

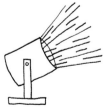
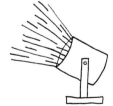

Trace the hands of as many people
as possible HERE:

CREATING YOUR V.I.P. STAND UP SET:

Answer the following questions to discover your best joke material!

Things that are unique about me (hobbies, friends, family, interests):

"I grew up with six brothers. That's how I learned to dance- waiting for the bathroom."

~Bob Hope

Things that make me really excited:

"I like fruit baskets because it gives you the ability to mail someone a piece of fruit without appearing insane. Like, if someone just mailed you an apple you'd be like, "Huh? What is this?" but if it's in a fruit basket you're like, 'This is nice!'"

-Demitri Martin

Joke ideas:

Things that worry me:

"Isn't it a bit
unnerving that
doctors call
what they do
'practice?'"
  -George Carlin

Things that frustrate or confuse me:

"I hate false
advertising, like
'Skittles: taste
the rainbow.'
No one's ever
been like, 'Rainbow,
right you guys?'"
  -Amy Schumer

Joke ideas:

OBSERVATIONS:

keep track of funny, weird, or interesting
things you notice daily!

Turn some of your observations into jokes:

Hide these notes where a member of your entourage will find them and watch his/her reaction!

I just wanted to let you know, sir, that I regrettably stole a blade of grass from your front lawn. My apologies!

I know you are a movie star disguised as a nurse in order to prep for your movie role. Your secret is safe with me! xoxo - -your biggest fan

---

Make your own:

Make your own:

Picture Telephone

A dog walker dancing with a pop star in a hurricane.

Draw a silly event below:

On the next page have a member of your entourage caption your picture by guessing what it is!

A picture of _____

Show another member of your entourage the previous caption and ask him/her to draw a picture of it below:

Show someone only the picture on this page and have him/her caption it on the next page:

A picture of _____

Show someone only the caption on the previous page and have him/her draw the final picture below:

See how your original picture changed!

SCAVENGER HUNT #3
CREATE A MASTERPIECE!

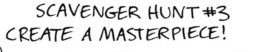 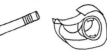   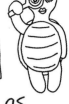

Find as many of the following items as possible and then build/create something with the materials!

- A glove
- Cotton balls
- Rubberband
- A very shiny penny
- 6 paper clips
- a toilet paper roll
- 7 sheets of toilet paper
- 2 scrunched up paper towels
- a bandage
- a page from a newspaper
- Hospital menu
- A pencil
- Straw
- Foil
- Lid for coffee cup
- A disposable cup
- Empty potato chip bag
- Medical mask
- Crackers
- Adhesive tape
- Gauze
- Sticky notes

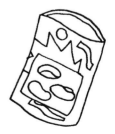

Vent your negative feelings:

Design your own Hospital Bracelet:

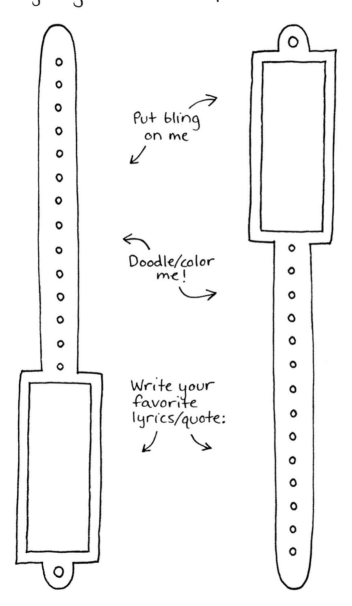

Put bling on me

Doodle/color me!

Write your favorite lyrics/quote:

WORDS TO IMPRESS #2:

"Evil witches in fairy tales often have lots of **verrucas!**"

Xerostomia: (zero **sto** mee ah) dry mouth

Xerosis: (zi **row** sis) dry skin

Epistaxis: (ep uh **stack** sis) nose bleed

Odontalgia: (oh don **tal** gee uh) toothache

Singultus: (sing **gull** tus) hiccup

Sternutation: (sturn u **tey** shun) sneeze

verruca: (ver **roo** ca) wart

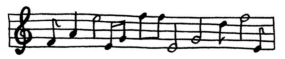

Write a rap, poem or song about how you're feeling today:

TIC TAC TOE:

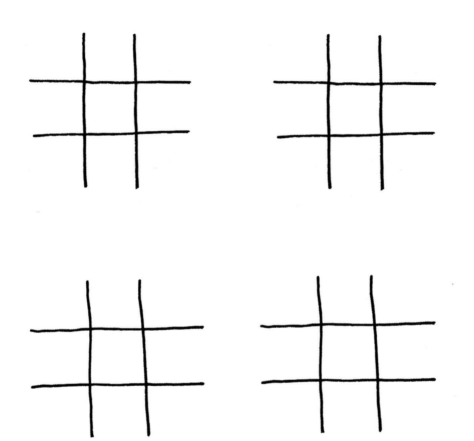

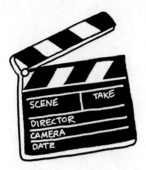

MY LIFE IS...

A soap opera because:

A reality show because:

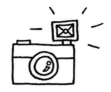

The Paparazzi Wants Pictures!

TAKE PHOTOS OF YOU AND YOUR ENTOURAGE:

☐ Performing a cool dance move

☐ Wearing sunglasses

☐ Dressed up as twins

☐ Creating your own handshake

☐ Posing for the Red Carpet

Inspirational Quotes:

"I've heard there are troubles of more than one kind. Some come from ahead and some come from behind. But I've bought a big bat. I'm all ready you see. Now my troubles are going to have troubles with me."
— Dr. Seuss

"It's kind of fun to do the impossible."
— Walt Disney

"I've learned that people will forget what you said, people will forget what you did, but people will never forget how you made them feel."
— Maya Angelou

"The best way to cheer yourself up is to try to cheer somebody else up."
— Mark Twain

MAKE UP YOUR OWN:

Collect doodles from others:

V.I.P. Knowledge:

If someone has to be in the hospital for the same reason as you, what advice would you give him or her?

Rip out this page,
make it into a ball
and PLAY!

V.I.P. PRESS

Words and phrases that the press can use when they write about you!

PLAY PSYCHOLOGIST:

Ask members of your entourage what they see in each picture.

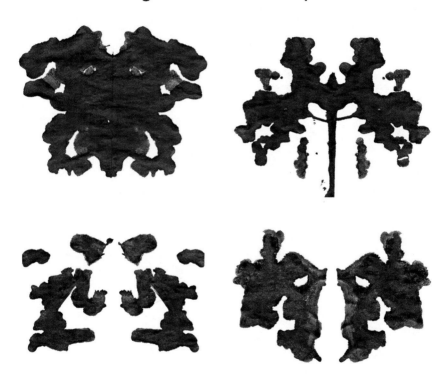

Weirdest answer:

Funniest answer:

Someone I agreed with:

DECODE THE MESSAGE:

"Promise me you'll always remember:
You're braver than you believe, and
stronger than you seem, and smarter
than you think."
—A.A. Milne

Write a message to someone in
MIRROR-LANGUAGE:

Make as many words as you can
with the letters in
I AM A VERY IMPORTANT PATIENT:

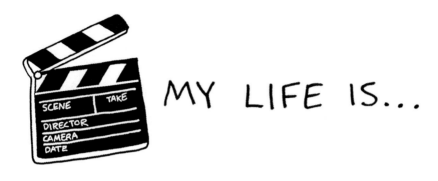 MY LIFE IS...

An action film because:

A viral YouTube video because:

Map out the things that fill your heart:

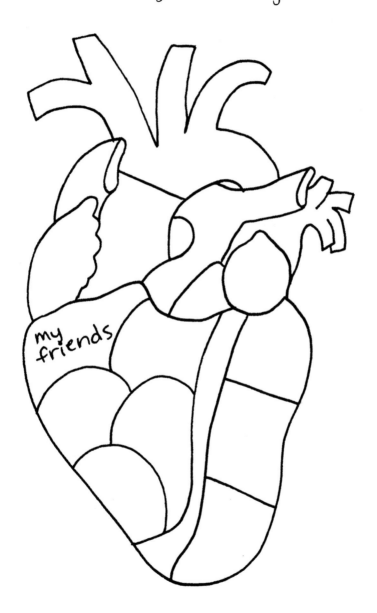

my
friends

Notes to inspire the people who make you
feel like a VERY IMPORTANT PATIENT:

To:
From:

You're the best
because...

To:
From:

To:
From:

To:
From:

Write a wish over and over:

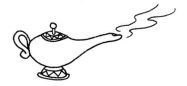

WHAT'S UP DOC?

- -

MEMOS FOR MY ENTOURAGE

For my:
- ☐ Doctor
- ☐ Nurse
- ☐ Other; _____
_____

Concerning:
- ☐ Questions I have
- ☐ Comments
- ☐ Ideas
- ☐ Problems
- ☐ Something else

- -

MEMOS FOR MY ENTOURAGE

For my:
- ☐ Doctor
- ☐ Nurse
- ☐ Other; _____
_____

Concerning:
- ☐ Questions I have
- ☐ Comments
- ☐ Ideas
- ☐ Problems
- ☐ Something else

WHAT'S UP DOC?

MEMOS FOR MY ENTOURAGE

For my:
- ☐ Doctor
- ☐ Nurse
- ☐ Other; _____
_____

Concerning:
- ☐ Questions I have
- ☐ Comments
- ☐ Ideas
- ☐ Problems
- ☐ Something else

MEMOS FOR MY ENTOURAGE

For my:
- ☐ Doctor
- ☐ Nurse
- ☐ Other; _____
_____

Concerning:
- ☐ Questions I have
- ☐ Comments
- ☐ Ideas
- ☐ Problems
- ☐ Something else

WHAT'S UP DOC?

MEMOS FOR MY ENTOURAGE

For my:
- ☐ Doctor
- ☐ Nurse
- ☐ Other;_____
_____

Concerning:
- ☐ Questions I have
- ☐ Comments
- ☐ Ideas
- ☐ Problems
- ☐ Something else

MEMOS FOR MY ENTOURAGE

For my:
- ☐ Doctor
- ☐ Nurse
- ☐ Other;_____
_____

Concerning:
- ☐ Questions I have
- ☐ Comments
- ☐ Ideas
- ☐ Problems
- ☐ Something else